Diagnosis:
CANCER

I Can't Be Here

E L A I N E   U O N E L L I

PAGE PUBLISHING, INC.
New York, NY

First originally published by Page Publishing, Inc. 2018

ISBN 978-1-64214-811-4 (Paperback)
ISBN 978-1-64214-812-1 (Digital)

Printed in the United States of America

2019

May you be blessed as you
read this book.

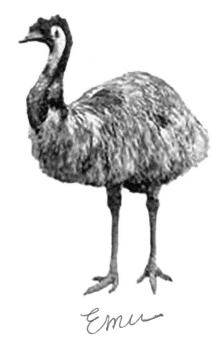

Emu

Elaine (Martin) Uonelli

Guided by God on this journey with faith, hope, and courage when my life took an unexpected turn in the road and I came face-to-face with cancer.

In memory of my beloved husband, Dr. Anthony R. Uonelli—without him and his love, support, and influence, this cross in the road would have been more difficult.

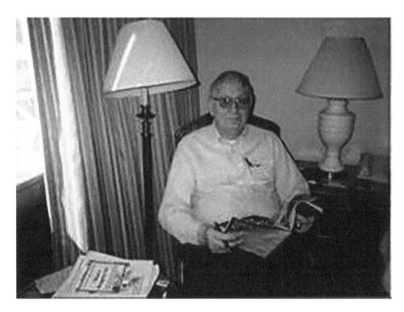

my husband, Dr. Anthony R. Uonelli

Dedication

T his book is dedicated to every person who has had any connection with cancer. It's a tribute to their indomitable spirit and their stalwart will. Sustained by faith and hope, survival and victory are their goals. God bless you and give you strength.

Contents

Prologue

In life you can make your own choices; for instance, not to get on a plane or not to eat that second piece of cake. You are in control and you know what you want and how to achieve it. When cancer comes into your life, your choices are not your own, and you don't have control anymore. You can't run from cancer or hide from it. You can say I don't want cancer, but it's not your choice; it is the cancer's choice whom it picks and when and how. Once it picks you, it is part of your surroundings and every breath you take. It controls your path in life and is now in control of your destiny.

The battle is between you and cancer, and cancer is your enemy. You no longer breathe to live; you breathe to survive. The invasion you feel happening to you is confusion, helplessness, and loss of control.

You look to God for answers even if you were not spiritual before. You are not praying for the well-being of others; you are now praying for yourself. You ask to be given strength and guidance in this battle.

You ask God to stand next to you on this battlefield for cancer is the devil. He is quick and sly and will be merciless in this fight. Yes, you may have your spouse, family, and friends, but they cannot help you in this battle.

Cancer has no boundaries. It will give you ups and downs, highs and lows. It is sneaky and will give you hope at times. You cannot banish the danger of cancer, but you can banish the fear. God will give you strength. He will help you confront your fears and fight the beast within. He will guide you with His love so that you have the will to conquer this evil. You know you have a harsh and cruel road to travel, but with faith and hope, you can face this challenge.

Introduction

I had the usual childhood diseases before all the vaccines. I would be considered a healthy woman by any standard.

Cancer happens to others, not to the likes of me. The dreaded cancer diagnosis affects countless people throughout the world. Those untouched are fortunate. Their contact is through the media, literature, art, poetry, and song. They are the spectators. When a family member, a close friend, or an acquaintance is afflicted, the separation lessens. As victims, we become active participants.

Twenty days after my sixty-seventh birthday, I was diagnosed with Burkitt-like lymphoma (Burkitt-like lymphoma rather than true Burkitt lymphoma because something was off in my DNA blood work.)

This is my story.

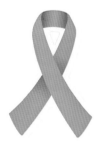

The Mass

The morning of February 4, 2008, I awoke with a sizeable swelling on the left side of my neck that inhibited movement down and to the left; it was very tender to the touch. I also noticed a slight scratchiness on the left side of my throat. I asked my husband, Anthony, who is a private practice doctor, to check out the enlargement. At first he wanted to have my dentist and an ENT specialist examine the growth. We decided to wait a few days to see if the condition worsened. The swelling seemed to go down as days went by.

On February 21 I went for a routine appointment with my primary care physician (PCP) for blood pressure monitoring. He listened to my update, checked my neck, and prescribed ten days of antibiotics.

I returned to my PCP's office on March 3. The size of the swelling had decreased slightly but was not resolved. My husband requested an additional ten days of the antibiotic regimen since there was some improvement. The doctor also drew blood for a full-panel analysis at my husband's request.

March 10 found me back at the PCP's office. Anthony and my doctor decided to have an ENT specialist see me. Anthony pleaded to expedite the appointment, and my primary complied. He called the office; they would work me in. I left the office with requisitions for a mammogram, a chest X-ray, and a CT scan of the neck.

The ENT's receptionist gave us a few pages of questions that my husband filled out for me. Although the waiting room was very busy, we did not have to wait long before the doctor saw us.

The initial questions posed by the doctor were, first, "Do you have a cat?" and, second, "Have you ever smoked?"

First the manual/visual look-see. Fingers in the mouth, under the tongue, and just about everywhere triggered the gag reflex. Yuck! Then the doctor sprayed a topical anesthetic up the nose and down the throat to enable him to check these areas fiber-optically—a horrible experience. Enough said, for I cannot begin to describe the sensation.

Last was an injection of anesthetic to prepare the neck for the needle biopsy. The ENT took specimens from three different sites and wrote orders for a CT scan with contrast.

Unbeknown to me, Anthony had considered the possibility of Hodgkin's disease—that spells the imminent *death knell* for sure. No wonder he had an anxious look and demeanor. I mentioned mumps—I had them on one side the summer following kindergarten.

After the question about cats, my spouse researched cat scratch fever. It would be wonderful if the etiology of my problem were so simple, but the contemplation of disposing of our family cats, Symphony and Domino, would be heartbreaking.

March 5. The medical campus is large, and we were lucky to find a parking space near one of the entrances. I checked in at the desk and had another questionnaire to complete. I had preregistered my insurance info over the telephone—they needed to know I was covered and they would get paid.

The mammogram was first. After the procedure I was directed to a small waiting area in the hallway. While there I had a pleasant chat with a former Spanish teacher who was waiting to go in for her appointment. One of the nurses took me to another area, where she inserted a needle to establish a line for injection of the dye contrast. First she tried the elbow bend on the inside of my arm—no luck. She then went to the top of my right hand and finally got a vein. She added a saline solution to determine if the fluid would go in and out. The CT technician was not satisfied with the needle placement. She went halfway down my left inside forearm, seeking a cooperative vein—it seemed to take forever, but at last, the needle was placed satisfactorily. When the solution was injected there was a flood of warmth in my lower extremities. I was a little dizzy when I sat up, but I was soon OK.

Only one more test—hurrah, the end is in sight. The technician finished a chest X-ray and left to check on whether or not she might need to redo it. I requested bathroom privileges. Uh-oh, red splotches dotted my forehead, cheeks, and chin. Now what? When the woman returned, I remarked, "I suppose these red splotches are to be expected after an IV contrast study."

"No," she replied. She took me to another area for someone to look at my hives.

In the meantime, Anthony had been waiting over two hours and was getting anxious. He sent the receptionist to look for me. When she found me, she directed my spouse to where I was waiting. The radiologist looked at my rash and asked if I had a problem with itching. Fortunately, I could say no. He recommended Benadryl if itching should become a problem. My husband asked if he had checked the CT reading; he said he was in the process of doing so and invited Anthony to go back with him (physician-to-physician courtesy). More time passed, and my husband appeared with a diagnostic sheet in hand. Based on the image findings, the diagnosis looked like Warthin tumor—benign. My husband was relieved, but I won't feel home free until "the fat lady sings" as the saying goes.

My arms looked as though I were a druggie. Three bruised areas on my left arm announced the needle punctures. The area on my right hand had only a pinprick dot. In the late evening, I had some itching on my legs and took a Benadryl.

Headaches continue to plague me—so much that I resorted to Tylenol with codeine. I can't help but think the headaches relate to the tumor. I am relatively pain-free when standing. In analyzing the problem, I concluded there must be pressure exerted on the nerves; when I sat—the head was at a different angle. When I add support behind the neck to raise my head I usually get some relief. I also have a flexible neck pillow to fit around my neck when in a prone position. I pity the folk who suffer constant pain; I don't think I could endure it.

On St. Patrick's Day we returned to the ENT's office, hoping for some answers. A biopsy should provide definitive information, but the report came back as inconclusive. Back to square one. The doctor rechecked nose, throat, and ears, which appeared okay. He performed another needle biopsy to send to the Cleveland Clinic cytology department. He said the mass could be parotid (salivary gland) or lymph—malignant or benign. He sent me to his associate for a second opinion.

This office, within the same building, was packed. They managed to work me in, but we had a long wait. The second doctor looked down my throat and felt my neck and under my arms.

Anthony was not present during the initial exam, but he had a brief conference with both doctors. Now we had to wait another week to find out what the Cleveland Clinic had to say.[1]

On March 18 God gave me a wake-up call.

I had been depressed about the lump in my neck, concerned by its visibility. We were at the pool at a local resort and saw a precious little six-year old girl. She had a growth the size of a goose egg dangling from her neck, and her hair was patchy and thin.

Although the child was grotesque to look at, I knew she was a fellow human being and made a point of saying hello. She readily responded and commented she liked my suit.

Who knows what this little girl has had to endure in her short life? I could not question her father in front of her—that would have been insensitive. I thought, how dare I bemoan my state in the face of her affliction. I believe God was reinforcing the blessings I have and was letting me encounter the plights of others as an object lesson.

March 24. It was hard to believe another week had passed. Time to review the second biopsy. The pathology report confirmed atypical lymphocytes, pointing to a diagnosis of lymphoma and ruling

---

[1] "All scripture is given by inspiration of God, and is profitable for doctrine, for reproof, for correction for instruction in righteousness" (2 Timothy 3:16).

out a parotid tumor. The doctor assured us this finding was on the positive side, for what I had was treatable and curable. Once again he did a cursory exam and checked areas containing lymph nodes—armpits, groin, etc. Everything appeared normal. The next step was a tissue biopsy—a piece of the mass is removed, frozen, and sent to the lab for an immediate reading to determine what kind of tissue they were dealing with.

On March 27 we went to the Medical Campus for the tissue biopsy. The Staff was friendly and helpful. The young woman who placed the needle for the IV took particular pains to tap out a visible vein on the top of my right hand.

Anthony was permitted to sit with me while I waited. My ENT doctor had many procedures in the morning and was running late. We checked in at 11:00 a.m. for the preliminary workup; the surgery was scheduled for 12:15 p.m. To pass the time, we read our individual books.

The anesthesiologist spoke with us prior to the surgery. She explained her role and what I could expect. Amazingly, I was unaware the anesthesia was being introduced—I just went to sleep. The next thing I knew, I was being awakened.

The women in the room chatted with me as they went about their duties. Then a woman dressed in ordinary clothes came up to me and said she was sorry, but they had found cancer. She spoke of attitude playing a big part where healing was concerned and said to think of the good cells attacking and destroying the cancer cells—and then she was gone. Who was this woman? Was she real or a figment of my imagination? After she left I felt as though I were wrapped in a warm security blanket and had no fears about the future.

I was a bit wobbly but I made it to the recovery room with assistance, where Anthony joined me. We were not given a conclusive diagnosis at that time.

I was feeling some discomfort, and the nurse gave me a couple of pills that took care of the pain. I left with a drain and a huge compression bandage over the incision.

On March 28, we entered the merry-go-round phase.

An appointment with my ENT proved to be somewhat traumatic. When he placed the drain, he inadvertently attached it to one of the deep sutures. I yelled when he tried to cut it out. At that point he asked my spouse to leave the room as he felt it would be hard on him to witness the ensuing procedure. I'm sure Anthony could have handled it, but he acquiesced to the doctor's request. After some pinches from a needle to inject a local anesthetic, the drain was removed painlessly.

With my husband back in the room, the doctor said I would need a PET scan which, in conjunction with the CT scan, would be more definitive. He also scheduled me to see an oncologist.

After we arrived home, my ENT called; he had been conversing with the oncologist concerning the aggressive growth of the tumor. They wanted me admitted to UH in Cleveland right away. Many calls were made on my behalf to make arrangements. UH called when they had a bed ready.

I suggested Anthony get someone to go with us. Previously he said he didn't need anyone. Well, when it came right down to it, he discovered he could use some company. Thankfully, a friend was available.

It was tricky finding the hospital because the road was torn up and there were many detours. At last we arrived and checked in at admitting. They were expecting me and only needed the usual paperwork.

Enter the Alien Land

I find myself disconnected from the world I know. I am thrust into alien territory.

My First Night

A bouncy young nurse with a pleasant manner looked after me.

The night shift doctor checked me over and asked many questions.

I have no medical history to speak of.

I was sad to see hubby go. He said he probably wouldn't be in the next day—understandable, but he did get a chance to meet the night doctor before leaving which was good.

The first order of business was to establish an IV line. Some veins are compliant while others are noncompliant. Unfortunately, mine come under the latter category. After three individuals tried to get a vein, the final attempt accessed one on the inside wrist of my dominant left hand. Do you know how handicapping this placement is?

The duty nurse brought in two IV bags of fluids. It would take about twenty-four hours to get all the fluid into my system. The IV pole accompanied me on my frequent visits to the white throne. It was nearly 1:00 a.m., so I had best turn in. I imagined the day would start early.

Keeping the door to my room open helped me feel connected with the outside world. Perhaps I heard some things I should not be privy to, but who was I going to tell?

A voice in the night cried out "Help me, help me, it hurts" over and over again. Gentle assurance from staff attempted to reassure this agitated, confused state.

"He's on the bed pan." Much later, "Are you done? Okay."

Heard from the hall: "What's today's date?" Answer: "Today is the twenty-second."

I listened to coughing, gagging, flushing toilets, flipping papers, chartings on a clip board, and clicking, and like a fog horn in the night, there were distant beeps of IV monitors and louder more insistent sounds nearby.

I had to notify the nurse when the urine cap was full—it was necessary to measure intake. When the urine was emptied, the seat was occasionally left up. I was caught three times—what an unpleasant surprise. I tried to develop the habit of checking the seat before I sit.

Note: I finally realized I could empty the urine myself and record time and amount. After all, a nurse was unable to respond immediately to every beck and call, and when you have to go you have to go.

My first morning an aide took me for a walk around. She identified the floor designations. Section D, shaped low, was referred to as low pod—my room was located there.

Another section was referred to as the upper high pod. To say I was more than confused would be putting it mildly. Think of an octopus with its tentacles extended, and you have an idea of the hospital-floor setup. Patient rooms are the tentacles, and the secretary, nurses' station, and doctors' coordinating area make up the body. A walking area surrounds the body—I called it the quadrangle. This was where I would get my *exercise* and meet many people.

I was trying to establish a routine walking pattern around the room and avoid lying down unless I felt sleepy. Also drinking my water—what else was there to do?

If you've never tried to put on a hospital gown, you don't know what you're missing—it is quite a challenge. Once I got the opening to the back, I figured out the sleeve snaps. With a lot of experimentation, I finally managed to put on a gown without assistance. A small accomplishment for most, but a major step forward for me! Could I manage a repeat performance? I kept my fingers crossed. For a modicum of modesty, I was double gowned, one in back and one in front—how attractive is that! At least I was covered.

The First Week

During this period many tests were run to determine the diagnosis, stage the tumor, and establish a baseline.

Each day followed a general routine.

There was a wake-up call at 6:30 a.m. to draw blood.

At 7:00 a.m., a plethora of medications arrived. For one who hates taking pills, this was an ordeal—especially before breakfast.

There were periodic checks on vital signs—blood pressure, heart rate, oxygen level and recording urine output.

I notified the kitchen concerning breakfast, lunch, and dinner choices from the menu.

Housekeeping finished their duties at 8:30 a.m.

In between times I cleaned up as best I could with a limited range of motion.

The oncologist in charge of my case arrived at 9:00 a.m. He examined me and asked more questions. He told me I was diagnosed with Burkitt-like lymphoma; it is common in youngsters or people from Africa—Burkitt like because it is not notably associated with the Myc gene or EBV infection.

At this stage the signs are promising for a cure. "Is it something I did that I shouldn't? Or I didn't do something I should have?" I asked my oncologist.

"No," he replied. "It's just bad luck. This is a fast-growing, aggressive cancer. Without treatment the patient has three to four months to live. On the positive side, this particular lymphoma is treatable and has a 96 percent cure rate." He proceeded to outline the therapy regimen he followed—CHOP chemotherapy, first day as an outpatient for a three- to four-hour infusion, five days to receive prescribed doses of various chemo, and one day for a twenty-four-hour run of Methotrexate.

He set me up for a controlled study that employed an additional ingredient to eradicate some of the side effects from chemo. Thirteen pages of protocol and explanations followed, mind-boggling to say the least. Sadly, the study was not approved in time for my case.

As the doctor talked, he might have been speaking another language, for I understood little of what he said. How can you ask questions when you are totally lost? In time some of the foreign-sounding chemo drugs had a familiar ring, and I began to understand how the simple breakdown of treatment days could extend into weeks and months.

Two expressions I became familiar with were "There's always a choice" and "Change of plans"—in other words nothing is carved in stone. Flexibility and adaptability are required to help you accept what comes your way.

Two pressing issues involved the relevance of time. I have experienced irregularity throughout my life, and it was compounded in my present circumstances. Three days with no relief required a laxative, suppository, or enema, which must go through pharmacy. It took all day before an enema was approved; just before it arrived, I evacuated. Hallelujah!

During my second week in the hospital, Meghan administered an enema per my request—going on day 3 without a bowel movement. After Dulcolax and milk of magnesia, I got some relief, but I knew there was more up there. My body seemed to react on a time delay for some unknown reason. I swear the stool softener of my first week at UH didn't take hold until the week I was home—frequent loose stools but what a relief. I was warned that some meds may induce diarrhea accompanied by a sore rectum, but I'll still take that over constipation. To avoid further problems, a stool softener was added to my meds.[2]

---

[2] "For all have sinned and come short of the glory of God" (Romans 3:23).

Me and My Pole

A woman asked
If I'd named my pole;
She called hers Big Brother.

I gave the matter
Considerable thought,
Sifting through my choices.

Albatross first came to mind,
But no, our pole's our sidekick;
Alter ego—other self,
Maybe that will do.

AE, now that could work;
I'm still not satisfied.
A staff member looked aslant
And asked if he were straight.
I answered, "No," and he replied,
"You could call it Eileen."

I pondered his suggestion,
Unable to relate;
At last I had to ask . . .
"I lean," oh, now I get it!
How could I be so slow?

I thought and thought
The next few days,
And then the name sprang forth—
Sunshine, what a perfect choice,
For it can say a lot . . .

Heavenly sunshine,
Sunshine on my shoulder,
Sunshine on a cloudy day . . .
And now my search is ended.

Naming the IV pole gave it a personality, for it is my lifeline.

On March 30 I was unhooked from the IV—hurrah! You never fully appreciate freedom of movement until you are restricted.

After a refreshing shower, I felt like a human being. I donned a T-shirt and pajama bottoms—I didn't miss the hospital gown. The day began with a delivery of many pills, yuck! What an appetizer before breakfast!

At the present my diet specifies sodium-free—where's the flavor? I ordered an omelet with everything allowed; prune juice, tea, and a banana.

More blood drawn, two jabs—the gal told me they were limited to two tries. At least they don't turn you into a pin cushion.

An alarm signal emanated from the IV pump—the message read "IV infusion complete / blockage on patient side/ air in tube." That sounds reassuring, doesn't it? The nurse said this was not an uncommon occurrence, and the pump just needed to be reset.

I had an MRI of the chest and head; it took about thirty-five minutes. The areas being checked had what was called antennas placed over them; to me they resembled some of the Star Wars costumes. One pillow under the knees and another at the side offered support and a bit of comfort. You hold a bulb in case you need to stop the test for some reason. Earphones placed around the head allow you to hear breathing instructions for the chest phase. Numerous mysterious sounds issued from the machine. Holding my breath for thirty seconds, four times seemed interminable. When the dye went in for the head exam it felt like needles and shredded glass entering my veins. The tech said I must have sensitive veins.

At 4:15 p.m. another team member came in to say she ordered a panoramic X-ray of my teeth to ensure no infection was present in the gums. This X-ray proved to be the easiest test of all to date. I heard "Hold your breath," no forewarning, and proceeded to follow directions. After nearly exceeding my limit, I discovered these directions were for a patient in another room.

Anthony called after I finished eating. I previously made a list of things to bring from home. He said everything was ready to bring in the next day.

I filled him in on what had transpired so far. I worry about his emotional state although he puts on a brave front for me; I try to do the same for him.

March 31 at 2:40 a.m. found me in a deep sleep. Suddenly I felt a flood of warmth; fortunately, I'd worn a pad to bed as a precaution against *accidents*. The aide was a love and said this was not an unusual occurrence. Hopefully, I won't have a repeat performance. With fresh gown and bedding, I returned to bed. On the bright side, I wasn't hooked up. I was giving thanks for small blessings.

At 6:20 p.m. a phlebotomist came in to draw seven tubes of blood. She applied heat and voila, using a syringe and applying some pressure, it was a successful draw, the gentlest yet. I wish I had her every time. At 6:40 p.m. I was weighed, and the night nurse came in to draw more blood. Four jabs this time and a blown vein with little success. She tracked down the phlebotomist.

Husband called to see what was happening. When he is not able to come to the hospital, he makes frequent calls—at all hours. How I love this man!

The bed was amazing. Although narrow, it had some type of mechanism that adjusted to the body contours—a miracle that soothes the back. Overhead was an air exchange that emitted cool air, a bit chilly at times, but I covered my nose and wore socks. Anthony was bringing my afghan, which never failed to keep me warm.

I really try to be religious about drinking water. I know it's important to keep hydrated, certainly preferable to IV fluids.

I had finished breakfast when my team arrived. They acquainted me with upcoming diagnostic tests. I intended to do my morning ablutions after returning my tray, but transport was waiting to take me down to nuclear medicine for the MUGA, a test for the heart. Two jabs to draw more blood for this procedure. The test checks the left ventricle to ensure it is functioning properly and to determine the heart is strong enough to withstand the onslaught of chemo. Time out while they check the blood. Next comes the dye inserted into the IV; it hurt just like the MRI dye. More waiting. We moved into a room housing a behemoth machine. Arms had to be raised over the head for twenty-five to thirty minutes to complete the test, *torture*! Now what? Something malfunctioned in the cameras. At least I could put my arms down. The cameras still weren't working given a second try. After more downtime they were finally able to complete the test.

On to another room for the PET scan. Once again arms had to be raised over the head for thirty-five minutes. More torture!

In between tests I made bathroom visits as often as I could—all that water, you know.

By the time I got back to my room, my spouse and a friend were waiting. Anthony appeared pale, and it looked like his back was hurting him, although he tried to hide it. He brought all the things I requested, bless his heart. Even though they had been waiting a long time, they stayed to visit.

Parting from my husband was heartrending. We tried to be strong for each other, but our emotions got the better of us. Anthony called when he got home; it is always a relief to hear he made it home safely. It is close to an hour's drive one way.

He said he called Betty and invited her over for coffee. She was eighty-seven years old, a dear woman and such a trooper.

A bit later my violin teacher called to wish me well. She would come to see me if she got the chance.

I selected some DVDs to watch. It wasn't long before my head started to hurt. Beth, my night nurse, gave me Tylenol when I called. She attempted to flush my IV stem, and it elicited the same pain as the dyes. She said that wasn't right, examined the area, and decided to remove the IV plant as I wouldn't need it that night. Another insertion would take place tomorrow in the morning—hopefully it would be better. I should not be having all that discomfort when other agents were flushed into the tube.

Amy called Mary to replace the IV. She got it on the first jab— the inside of my right wrist hurt like hell. We weren't promised a "rose garden," were we?

Mary drew blood on April 1. Phenomenal! One barely perceptible prick and she was in. "Can I hire you to draw all my blood?" I begged.

"I've been asked that before," she acknowledged.

I'll not keep repeating vital signs and medications for they are ongoing; however, the previous night I received a pill to protect my kidneys from invasion of what is to come.

My soul mate called around 9:00 a.m.; he was planning to come in with Betty.

Oh no, they had to find another IV site as this one also elicited pain on infusion.

The team arrived at 9:30 a.m. and discussed test results so far. It appeared that the cancer was localized in one small lymph node. Am I blessed or what? There were more tests on the docket, and then we would know the whole story.

At 10:30 a.m., Mary successfully placed the IV needle—hurrah! I hoped this one was a winner.

I managed to walk ten times around the quadrangle—a record for me. Ha!

Katrina hooked me into fluids; all was calm on the western front. Relaxing medication was added to the IV in preparation for the bone marrow sample removal, which was done in the room—no problem.

During one of his visits, Anthony ran into the music therapist. She had her guitar and a keyboard. He invited her into my room so we could meet. Each time I was in the hospital, I notified her so she could add me to her schedule.

My husband suggested I call Gretchen, our longtime friend, and give her an update. She was shocked by the news. She promised she and her husband would keep in touch with Anthony. I also talked to Cathy, and she said she would send her son Chris to work with my husband; their family would be supportive.

The day nurse awakened me and said my team would be there shortly. I no sooner finished in the bathroom when they arrived. They reported that everything looked good to this point, and I may require fewer rather than more treatments to knock this thing. Now that's good news!

I'd had nothing to eat or drink since midnight, pending placement of a permanent chest port that went under the skin.

Anthony called for an update. He said he sent me a card, and it took him forever to address the envelope. He is such a sweetheart!

Not to be redundant, but I am so blessed. God has been good to me and brought me through many adversities.

I now know that nurses' aides are called clinical partners. I cannot keep up with all the titles!

Around 11:00 a.m. a resident arrived to discuss the port placement procedure. Anthony called when he was here and spoke to him. Our neighbor Gail called and wished me well. She said my husband seemed to have it all together when he talked with her husband for an hour.

The transport team arrived to take me to surgery. The next thing I knew, it was nearly 6:00 p.m. I was alert and talkative as usual. The phone was ringing when I got back to the room—it was Cathy. We talked for nearly an hour. I had just hung up when Anthony called.

He had been trying to get through for two hours. Poor hubby. I was able to assure him that all was well.

I called the kitchen for something to eat; they still had me listed as no food. My nurse had to call and remove the restriction. I called the desk and waited—as if I couldn't afford to miss some meals! At last food service contacted me and asked what I wanted.

I couldn't figure out how to get into my gown with the IV line in place, and I was freezing. My night nurse resolved this dilemma.

Decision—needle placed in port tonight or wait until the wee hours. I opted for the next day in order to give the surgery site a chance to adjust. A nurse brought in a second pillow.

Headache is troublesome; my nurse gave me two Oxycodone pills. They took a while to kick in but did wonders when they did. Husband called around 1:00 a.m. He had just arrived home from the local resort after a hot tub workout and a stop at a nearby restaurant for a bite to eat.

An early-morning nurse arrived to place the needle in the port. Rats, she met with resistance. The surgeon inserted a double port, and his placement was deep—lucky me; just think, if I were skinny, he couldn't have gone so deep. The nurse probed to find the port access. I hadn't realized it required a needle through the skin. What was I thinking?

The area was tender and slightly swollen. After two tries a second nurse was called in.

She acknowledged it was difficult to isolate the port. She inserted a needle and feared it had not taken. Success at last—the port was flushed. We were not done yet; there was still another needle to insert.

The doctor in charge of my case arrived to explain the treatment plan. Chemo must be injected into the spinal column (a lumbar puncture) to protect the brain from invasion, or they shave the head and establish a port under the skin to introduce chemo in small quantities. Nine lumbar punctures did not sound appealing, and I opted for the Ommaya. A doctor from neurology stopped in to explain the procedure.

The entire Powell family came to visit and brought a beautiful red cape—just what I needed to keep my top half cozy warm. The time passed all too quickly. This whole thing is so hard on my dear husband. I wish there were some way I could spare him. He's used to being in control of situations, and this has left him feeling helpless.

Headache in the wee hours, but two Tylenol took care of it—had a good night.

Blood drawn at 6:00 a.m. through the port was a welcome relief from vein intrusion.[3]

I wrote a poem called "Invasion." I wanted several copies of it. The secretary was off duty, and I left it at the desk. The following day the dear woman left the copies outside my door. Mind you, she was up to her eyeballs and beyond with her regular duties and other copying jobs, yet she made time for me. Bless her heart.[4]

---

[3] "For the wages of sin is death" (Romans 6:23a).

[4] "For God so loved the world that He gave His only begotten Son, that whosoever believeth in Him should not perish, but have everlasting life" (John 3:16).

Invasion

A lump appears,
Biopsies done,
Malignant or benign?
    What is our fate?
    What is our course
    When cancer's diagnosed?
Why me? I do not ask,
For who am I
'Mongst countless others?
    Teams of doctors
    Join our fight
    To overthrow disease,
    Rally our defenses,
    Bring out the ammunition . . .
    Radiation? Diet? Pills?
    Chemotherapy?
Treatable and *curable*—
Words we trust and cling to.
Untreatable and *terminal*—
Words we dread to hear.
    See us walking in the halls,
    Pushing IV poles;
    Our foe does not discriminate—
    Attacks both young and old.
    Respects not color, rich or poor,
    Politics or gender . . .
    Not for wimps, our hearts cry out
    As we move along.
We form our own community,
V our vict'ry sign,
Unbowed we move along;
All are equal here.

Nurses and assistants,
Staff and all who share
Our burdens and our care;
Treasured beyond measure,
Without them we'd despair.
Support from loved ones, family, friends
Lends strength and buoys spirits;
It's good to know we aren't alone . . .
Forever and beyond.

God bless you all.

Looking forward to a bald head—not! At least the hair-washing issue was resolved. If a person has any vain tendencies, she can leave them outside the door. With no hair, especially for a woman, much of the physical individuality is lost. You can tell I am preparing myself for this eventuality.

Husband called around noon for the latest update from my team encounter.

I received a steroid given twenty-four hours in advance of the CT scan of the head, which was scheduled for some time the following morning. The steroid left an unpleasant taste in my mouth; I chewed some gum to offset the effects.

I was learning to be prepared for changes in a plan. I had to have a second MRI of the head.

Someone from the neurology department came in to prep my head for the next day's surgery. He shaved off small patches of hair and used a skin marker to circle specific areas. He placed some type of button that resembled an alien eye. Maybe they're ETs in disguise, making implants for outer space tracking. I've watched too much sci-fi, haven't I?

I forgot to count the patches of *stuck-on eyes* and anticipated seeing bald patches, but the nurse expertly arranged my hair, so I hardly noticed the shaved areas. I requested they remove all my hair before surgery rather than having a gradual fallout. Besides, they were going to remove additional patches for the surgery. Doesn't going totally bald make perfect sense? A CT scan would follow the surgery.

At 6:40 a.m. I awoke with the need to pour out my heart to my spouse, words too difficult to say face-to-face. A letter, tearfully written, offered the catharsis I needed.

Transport arrived at 7:45 a.m., just as my team was making rounds. I already had two visits from representatives of neurosurgery to prepare me for what they were doing and what could happen—in layman's terms known as CYA ("cover your ass"). Please forgive my crudeness, but it is what it is.

I didn't realize a separate IV apart from the port entry had to be put in place. I am thankful I was out of it, so I don't know how much difficulty they had locating a vein.

I was unaware of drifting off. When I came to myself, I was grateful my brain was still functioning; I had been told I would probably have some memory loss and confusion. I read that every time you undergo anesthesia, you lose brain cells. I can't afford to lose too many more; the natural aging process takes enough.

Out of recovery and on for an MRI of the head to check out the port placement. This scan only took ten minutes—then back to my room.

Intubation and open mouth resulted in a sore throat and dry mouth. The nurse brought ice chips, which helped immensely. My voice was croaky and I needed lots of ice chips and water throughout the day.

I ordered breakfast and proceeded to wait. The nurse had verbally placed a POA (nothing to eat or drink) order withdrawal. Unfortunately, we failed to notice the sign was still posted outside the door, so no breakfast was dropped off. By the time I realized what had happened many hours later, I encountered a nurse who kindly placed my lunch/dinner order and recommended a fruit plate. I'm so glad I followed her advice—it was very good.

My husband continues to show strain, but he is trying to keep positive. It's too bad parking is such a bear. He said they had to walk the equivalent of two football fields before they got to my room. Somewhere along the line, he located a wheelchair for Betty. Truth be known, he could have used one himself, but he would never admit to it.[5]

---

[5] "For by grace are ye saved through faith: and that not of yourselves: it is the gift of God: not of works, lest any man should boast" (Ephesians 2:8, 9).

On Top of Old Baldy

On top of Old Baldy,
No hair on my head.
I'm going through chemo,
No more need be said.

I opted for full shave,
No fallout for me.
Became a true egghead,
As you plainly see.

Our beauty's from inside.
Don't look in the mirror.
Skin deep doesn't measure
Why we're really here.

A *V* stands for *vict'ry*,
A sign that we share.
We're fighting a battle
That few others dare.

We don't need your pity.
We don't need your tears.
We do need your love,
Your support, and your cheer.

Gail and Cathy call daily; thank God for special friends. The phone company is gaining a lot of additional revenue from the long distance calls. I know I'll drop over when *our* bill comes in, for Anthony calls five to eight times a day. He likes to be abreast of all the developments. Not to mention he really enjoys telephone conversations in general.

Little to report at the team visitation. Treatment should start Tuesday or Wednesday, depending on healing of head port.

The neurosurgery team said that everything went well. The surgeon removed my dressing and said to keep it dry. I was told the stitches were not to be touched; they would dissolve in three to four months.

I cannot believe how rested I feel after each interrupted space of sleep. In this alien territory, I am not the same lethargic individual who occasionally gets spurts of energy to accomplish what must be done and falls back into sloth.

I have yet to become adjusted to being tethered to the IV pump. My typical pattern is to start walking in one direction, think of something I need, and turn around, forgetting I am hooked up. The inevitable happened—the line disconnected from the tubing, and fluid was dripping out. I held the line up, oblivious to a free swinging line from my port, which was scattering a blood trail—what a mess!

At 12:30 a.m. nature called. Egad, somehow IV lines and cords from bed to pump were totally tangled. I made an effort to untangle and failed miserably. I've never been good at puzzles. This segment should have been videotaped—no doubt it would have received some attention on the world's funniest video. Thankfully, my backup bladder protection did its thing as I was trying to sort out the lines—it's a wonder I didn't knock over the pump as I was lifting the wheels to free up the tangle. I had to call for assistance twice; Dorothy came to my rescue and restored status quo.

Adjusting my position in bed at 2:30 a.m. and feeling all was right in the world when I felt wetness through the gown—yep, sprung a leak. When checked, somehow the dressing covering my port was off and the needle had pulled out. Nurse Katrina says we'll call it a mystery. That wasn't the greatest piece of news. Accessing this port has been a challenge from the get-go. Katrina literally made a stab for a port—no luck. I explained I'd been told they needed to use one-inch needles—of course, none were available on this floor, and they had to check other floors. In the meantime, I was maintaining pressure on the gauze pad over the port. "Don't go to sleep now," Katrina cautioned, which I was sorely tempted to do. Time passed, and Katrina returned, needles in hand. Okay, where to go?

Katrina felt with her fingers and said she would push the needle back through the last hole for starters. Hurrah, we had a winner. Flush and draw—success.

A period of good rest followed, and Anthony called at about 4:00 a.m. In the meantime, all labs were drawn and vital signs recorded.

I could feel the start of a canker sore in back of my tongue despite my efforts to follow the oral hygiene plan. I recall using silver nitrate sticks when in college. I had a nasty infection from vigorous brushing with stiff bristles and slipping up on the gum line. An ugly laceration resulted. The doctor said, "No toothbrush did that." Of course he had not witnessed the original event.

I am now aware of peripheral neuropathy in fingers and toes. I was warned this was a possible side effect from some of the drugs I received.

At 5:10 a.m. my bladder awakened me. Watch those lines, lady! Did I mention the hemorrhoids I managed to pop? I haven't been straining, honest.[6]

---

[6] "I can do all things through Christ which strengtheneth me" (Philippians 4:13).

Treatment

On April 7 I went home for a week and kept busy playing catch up. There is no place like home. One must follow hospital protocol every time one leaves, which includes a dismissal sheet with instructions and prescriptions. When you return to the hospital, you must be readmitted. I lost track of how many times we repeated this procedure.

April 16 was my first infusion as an outpatient. It took over an hour to get the needle placed and the chemical metered out in degrees to allow the body time to acclimate to the drug. Midway into the procedure I had a reaction—face felt hot and slightly itchy.

The technician stopped the drug and introduced counteraction to offset the symptoms. After a thirty-minute delay, they resumed the Rituxan infusion, which was completed without further incident. My dear husband focused on my face the remaining six hours to note any changes—a long day.

On April 17 Felicia called from admitting and said she would call back around noon. In the meantime, two pilots required a physical ASAP. I took a chance and told them to come in immediately. Felicia called and said they had a bed around 1:00 p.m. I explained my dilemma and said we should be there by three. Hurrying to transmit the FAA physical, load the car, and buck traffic, we made it to the Bowell building around four. Too late—Felicia had left, and we were directed to Lerner Tower Admitting to wait for another bed. They cannot hold a bed if emergencies arise. One young woman had been waiting since 1:00 p.m. In the meantime, the pressure buildup from my extended mass gave me a terrible headache—walking helped. A nurse said I could return to the Bowell building for medication.

During hospital stays the days followed a general routine. Blood draws usually took place after 6:00 a.m., and morning meds follow. The kitchen is notified to place breakfast order. After eating it is time to attend to personal needs, followed by a midmorning visit from my team to review lab results, explain upcoming procedures, and answer any questions I might have. Vital signs are taken throughout the day at various intervals. I try to walk around the quadrangle in the morning and afternoon for much-needed exercise.

On April 19 at 6:15 a.m., Devin came to draw blood. First prick did it—*hurrah!*

Megan came in at eleven and attempted to access the ports. Her one try was unsuccessful.

From 4:00–4:30 p.m., chemo infusion. I had to close my door to deaden the sound of a man vomiting—it was starting to make me feel sick. I wish I had a headset to help filter out unpleasant sounds.

Devon returned to draw more blood. The procedure did not go as smoothly this time; he had more difficulty locating the port; it really hurt.

My team was impressed over decreased size of the mass following the chemo treatment.

One horrible side effect of the chemo was a canker sore on my tongue and thrush. Although I could swallow, I was unable to chew or touch anyplace in my mouth. I can only describe it as having acid in your mouth. Pain medication was recommended, but it did not relieve the fire in my mouth, nor did it enable tongue movement without extreme discomfort. My medical team and nurse came up with various combinations to swish and swallow or to spit out. The relief was temporary, but it helped. Later I discovered that two pain pills relieved the burning and induced sleep. How does one evaluate pain? The scale my hospital used, which may be universal, is one to ten—the higher the number, the greater the degree of pain. I learned you don't have to suffer excruciating, intolerable pain to justify a pain pill. My team assured me I would not become addicted, for my prescriptions were a relatively low dose. Once again the time elements come into play. You ring for the nurse—you need relief *now*. Then you wait. I know I am not the only patient my nurse has; her tasks are multiple and must be prioritized. This fact does not help time pass faster for the waiting patient although the caregiver feels she has responded promptly.

Meghan brought in Teresa to try for port access—no dice even after they looked at original X-ray of placement.

At 12:15 p.m., Linda drew fluid for the bone marrow test. There was some bleeding, and she said she might have hit a tiny vein as platelets were still up. The injection went okay, and I was cleaned up with a fresh gown.

At 12:40 p.m., Meghan injected IPA to access draw from port. Checked back, some pink. At 1:10 p.m. still pink. At 1:45 p.m., the third go was the charm—hallelujah! How resistant the insertion and how yielding the withdrawal, thank you, God, for guiding Meghan's untiring pursuit of the port and continuous attempts to get the needle to draw.

Kerry accessed the port for the morning draw. Praise God once again. She told me the twenty-third Psalm was one of her dad's favorite passages—"The Lord is my Shepherd."

Marie, a clinical partner, put me last on her rounds, which gave us time to visit. She is a Virgo and shared many traits listed in *Goodman's horoscope of the stars*.

Our hospital caregivers are remarkable, their patience unending and their gentle reassurance to meet their patients' needs—emotionally, physically, whatever might arise.

On April 21 the day flew by. Welcome words from team members—I was responding to treatment without noticeable adverse side effects thus far. Their prophylactic precautions were doing their thing.

When Anthony visited he demonstrated his ingenuity by putting the multitude of items I requested on a wheelchair and transporting them from the parking garage to my room. He brought in a Nokia cell phone for me to use; I had to read up on it. I was surprised when I read the battery could last up to a week. Am I dating myself here?

Physical surroundings are important to me: a colorful afghan on the bed buoys the spirit. A touch of home looking at a favored picture of loved ones on the bedside table and available tablets and pencils to write when the spirit moves me. The cell phone readily connects to the outside world. A CD player provides music that relaxes me. Watching selected DVDs helps pass the time. A head cover is welcome to provide warmth for my bald head, and comfortable slippers to walk around are a must. A nearby address book, stationery, and stamps are available if I feel like writing letters. To help adjust to my surroundings, I covered the wall with beautiful cards I received.

I am grateful for extra services offered—music therapy held the greatest appeal. Talking to others on my walks made me part of a community rather than feel isolated on a desert island.

Because of the difficulty locating my ports, the team decided to initiate a port-dye contrast, which requires twenty-four hour prep due to my previous reaction to the dye. This study provides port views allowing visualization of needle placement. I faded in and out of consciousness during the procedure. As I have two ports, they first pulled out both needles and inserted fresh ones. It took three attempts before both needles showed in the window. Proper needle placement was confirmed by the dye contrast—the top port is accessible, but the bottom port isn't responding. My nurse says my port has its own individual idiosyncrasies—aren't I lucky? The peripheral IV line—in place for a while—started hurting big-time, so now it's out.

Sudoku helps pass the time while on the sitz bath that cleanses and relieves hemorrhoids. In general my husband feels puzzles are a waste of time, yet he surprised me with two sudoku books.

Nurses not only collect and measure urine output but now also collect the arrival of diarrhea—isn't life great? After one run-through with my nurses, I can manage the sitz bath and collections myself. Another challenge conquered.

I have mouth and lip lesions as a side effect of my treatment. The inside of my mouth feels as though an acid bath ran over it—inside cheeks and lips are swollen and inflamed, an inferno supersensitive to any kind of touch. I am unable to perform routine dental care other than swishing fluids around. Canker sores on the side of my tongue contributes to excruciating agony. Periodically, the tongue suctions against the tortured cheeks, and when the suction releases, new pain waves follow. I can go from zero pain level to a ten in seconds. The treating doctors recommended morphine. I contend that no pain drug douses this unrelenting flame. My mouth needs soothing and numbing. BMX, a combination of Benadryl, Maalox, and Xylocaine, offers temporary relief. Basic functions of eating—chewing, sucking, swallowing—have to be modified now. It is painful to chew with a sore tongue and inflamed mouth mucosa. Thankfully, the act of swallowing has remained intact; we take for granted involuntary actions. Doing what comes naturally no longer works; it is necessary to exert voluntary control to avoid painful repercussions from eating. There is increased risk of biting into upper and lower inner labial cheeks and bruising edematous sides of the tongue, which are also tender. Need cooling. I found that a gentle finger massage was soothing and offers temporary relief. When I told my team, they said a finger massage is bacteria laden, and I don't need to risk an infection. They suggested the following—Betadine swabs, but no, they are too harsh for a sore mouth. Glycerin swabs, similar to hemorrhoid gel, will offer some relief, and an oral wound rinse, typically used for radiation patients, was prescribed.

What can I eat? Puréed cream soups like celery, mushroom, and chicken, something you can slurp through your teeth. Broths are good but harsh on a sore mouth—slurp and swallow.

During mouth issues, talking is painful. Reading and TV help pass the time.

Exercises recommended—with teeth together and lips pulled back, inhale deeply and exhale fully (repeat ten times). Repeatedly puff cheeks in and out. Alternate the exercises a.m. and p.m.

Unfortunately, these activities dried out my mouth. The oral wound rinse is wonderful. Please keep it coming.

When doctors promised my mouth would be better, I was looking for instant healing. Not so—imperceptible gains have been made. Unless I chart them, I am hardly aware they are occurring. Flare-ups and mouth discomfort are precursors indicating it is time for the BMX. My nurse promised to have standby available but forgot. With the next flare up, I tried rinsing with water, which did not help. I prayed arrival of the BMX would be soon. Praise God—it came when I needed it. There is no such thing as coincidence.

One of our doctor friends paid me a visit and explained that as my WBC increases, the mouth will respond. He is collaborating with others for remote healing. I have no idea what this entails.

On May 4 my WBC was 0.5; on May 5 my WBC was 1.6. Something must be working!

Side effects—you name it, I probably got it.

I remain in my room for bathroom availability when laxatives are working. During this phase my exercise consists of getting up and down.

Does the right hand know what the left hand is doing in a place like this? Impossible! I can't keep track of my own comings and goings, and the hospital staff is expected to be aware of my individual needs. I don't envy them. The partner who took my vital signs returned with a urine-specimen bottle and obstetrical wipes to clean the area before peeing. I succeed in voiding all around the jar but finally managed to reach my goal. No one came to pick up the urine. When I inquired of the nurse, she said she had not been notified, nor was any reference made of it in the chart. In the latter part of the day, the same partner reappeared to check vitals. I mentioned the waiting sample, and he took it with him.

My nurse drew blood early in the morning. Later two members of the staff arrived to draw blood. I mentioned I had an operational port, and they said they would check with the nurse. I did not see them again. Apparently, there was some sort of mix-up, and they were unaware the nurse had drawn the blood. Note to self—we must never take anything for granted and not be afraid to speak up if something should appear amiss.

I am presently armed with all kinds of mouth care and am married to the porcelain goddess.

No sooner had new hair begun to grow than it started to fall out. I asked if my head could be shaved, and my clinical partner said it was not a good idea, but he introduced me to a shampoo cap. Whoever heard of a shampoo cap? It resolved my issues. I am so fortunate to live in modern times.

Personal remedies: A little petroleum jelly or Vaseline goes a long way to soothe a dry nose and ears. Sitz baths after BMs are soothing. Availability of puzzles or reading material helps the time pass.

On May 7 my team said I was good to go—I was packed and ready. Then the doctor came in with the nurse and said I could not go home after all. What a blow! The tears flowed. He explained that the creatinine level had raised alarmingly, indicating trouble with the kidneys. It is difficult to pull oneself out of the doldrums, but it serves no purpose to sink into depression.

While waiting for a kidney and bladder ultrasound, another patient was wheeled up. I asked the woman what she was there for— she was diagnosed with pulmonary hypertension. We talked until they took me to ultrasound. While I was waiting for transport back to my room, a man was wheeled up. I asked how he was doing. "Not so good. They have to take something out of my side," he said.

"That does not sound like fun," I reply.

"No," he answered. Even with my blurred vision, sans eyeglasses, I could tell he was in sad shape.

Great improvement in mouth, but canker sore still inhibits chewing.

I waited all evening for TED Hose (compression stockings) in my size and did not realize a clinical partner had placed them on the tray. After mouth care, I checked the bag and saw the larger size had arrived. I tried to follow the explicit directions on how to put them on. I actually *started* at the proper end, but when I had difficulty, I reconsidered and started the other end. I got my foot into the stocking, but the rest was dangling. A nurse came to my rescue. It was no easy task—she even landed on her behind in the process, but she got those stockings on me. Her comment was "Whew! That made me work up a sweat!" These stockings offer relief for swollen feet and legs. Thank you, sweet Jesus. The nurse said it was okay to keep TED hose on unless they became uncomfortable. Once on they feel good, but they are a bear getting into because of the tight fit.

Fortunately, I was not indisposed when my team came in—everything hinges on the creatinine level. The renal doctors reported on the kidneys. Normally, following chemo, the creatinine level is low and increases in gradual increments. Alas, my level spiked, which put the kibosh on going home.

The latest news is that tests still show an increase but in small amounts. They expect the level to plateau and begin a gradual drop until it gets to normal. The question is, when can I go home?

The massage therapist stopped in; she previously worked as an RN but took a class in the art of massage to soothe and relax her patients. She offered unscented or lavender lotion or oil. I chose lavender oil. All I can say is ahhh. It was very relaxing. The therapist gave advice about raising toes, holding and relaxing to help swelling go down. I mentioned rotating ankles, and she said that was good also.

One of the renal doctors stopped by and said it would take one to two weeks for the creatinine level to be normalized—providing the kidneys start doing their job. Contributing to the problem was all the saline fluid I had been given while continuing my blood pressure medicine. He said I should not dangle my feet and try to have my feet raised fifteen degrees higher than my head. My team doctor said the etiology of the creatinine level rise was multifactored.

In the meantime, my dear husband arrived with all the bills that came during my absence, an oversized business checkbook and bank statement. He helped with stuffing envelopes and adding address labels.

I will be a happy camper when the swelling in my feet and legs dissipates. Good to be untethered from Sunshine, my IV pole—she needs the break. Ha!

On May 28 I arrived at the outpatient lab at 10:00 a.m., but all spots were filled. At 12:25 p.m. a chair was open. First they gave me a couple of pills followed by the infusion.

On May 30 I expected to go to the Bowell building at noon, but they called around 9:00 a.m. and said there was a bed available. A mad dash ensued, and we hit the road. Once at the hospital, we had to wait for orders. A nurse accessed both ports and did the blood draw; on to Learner Tower, floor 7 this time. New staff members to meet—they gave me a warm welcome. An Ommaya injection was first, followed by the chemo mixture.

On May 31 chemo regimen continued at intervals—so far, so good. My doctor said they would follow the therapy plan, and I could possibly go home Tuesday.

On June 1 Ommaya injection went smoothly, constipation issues resolved with milk of magnesium the previous night and suppositories the following day—still on stool softener two times a day.

On June 2 chemo at 5:45 p.m.—prep delayed.

On June 3 a group of trainees in music therapy and their professor were visiting from Ohio University to observe and to participate in our program. We had a wonderful music sharing before noon. One young lady accompanied herself on the guitar and sang—she had written about prayer and her relationship to God. It was beautiful and meaningful—I wish I had the words.

On June 11 I finished second round of chemo. The Methotrexate infusion produced another side effect—low potassium and magnesium levels. Boosters and pills were added to the regular medications to normalize. I was given two more pints of blood, no canker sores this time, thank God, but inside of cheeks are puffy and tender—I can still chew. The ends of my fingers are numb and very sore. I have adjusted pen position to the base of the thumb guided between second and third fingers. It's all about adaptability.

On June 13 Methotrexate must be out of my system before I can go home. In addition the blood count needs to be within a given range—one day at a time. The Ommaya injection into the head port went smoothly.

I understand we have been having temperatures in the nineties with high humidity. Being in a controlled environment with AC is a plus, to be sure.

Although I haven't been nauseated, I don't have much of an appetite. I understand the medicine has something to do with this. I don't even like water but tolerate club soda.

My soul mate has been supportive throughout. He visits nearly every day and makes a gazillion telephone calls in a twenty-four-hour period—he wants to know how I am tolerating the chemo treatment and needs reassurance. I have no adverse effects from treatment or meds at the time of his last call. All his knowledge makes everything worse for him. Ignorance is bliss!

June 14. Today is Saturday. If it were Friday the thirteenth, I would have superstitions confirmed.

In the normal (is there such a thing?) course of events, we expect chemo to gradually flush out of the system and cells to rebuild. The hand soreness has dissipated. As I continued to swish and spit the sodium bicarbonate solution, my mouth condition worsened. I now have blisters inside my bottom lip and cannot use the sponge tooth cleaner for it feels like sandpaper and acid. In the morning, the doctor said I might be able to go home if my labs and blood count were acceptable. I encountered the doctor in the early afternoon., and she said the Methotrexate level wasn't dropping like it should; in fact, there was a slight rise. And so I would be there at least another day. Two or three seems more likely to me—what a kick in the gut.

At 6:00 p.m. the renal team came to discuss the danger of toxicities from Methotrexate remaining in my system. I have none of the signs such as headaches and joint pain. The body must rid itself of conflicting antibiotics and resume normal functioning—the waiting game.

On July 16 I have had two hospital stays on the sixth floor and two on the seventh floor. I couldn't help but wonder what room would be available for my last round. A return to the sixth floor with the same nurse I had on the first admission—coincidence?

Under pressure to eliminate as much fluid as I was being given, it seemed there was little output and no feeling of urgency—unusual for me. Because of past problems, I feared the kidneys were slacking off. I forced down glass after glass of water and was rewarded at last. Frequent trips to the throne room can be inconvenient, but it's a relief to know my system is flushing out.

July 17. How things change. Forget about repeats—different issues arise all the time. I received two units of insulin because of elevated glucose and magnesium.

My team keeps on top of any potential threat, which is a good thing. They changed my pump, and there were four channels to deal with. What a program-procedure nightmare. The quality control tech and the nurse made a successful change over.

On July 18 Methotrexate was completed at 3:50 a.m. And again the waiting game begins—dealing with side effects as they arise. Added Lasik because output does not match intake. Two units of blood to compensate for lower hematocrit.

July 22. "What's wrong with me?" How feeble we human beings are. If only this problem were remedied, I would be satisfied. Oh no, now another dragon has arisen! How to equate discomfort levels?

Completing the last part of my third round of treatment, I have a comparison basis. As bad as things are with the immune system totally bottomed out, it's time to count my blessings.

August to September winding down.

The third round of chemo was not without side effects and complications. This time my blood counts were slow to normalize, which extended my hospital stay. Because of all the dextrose IVs, my sugar levels were elevated, so they gave me insulin and were keeping tabs on it. I'm thankful I'm not diabetic.

I've had my share of potassium pills. They are huge; even split in half, they are hard to get down.

Finally, on August 1, 2008, my blood levels were satisfactory. I was no longer neutropenic and was good to go home. The beginning of the following week, I was an outpatient—port flush and blood drawn. The lab results were satisfactory.

I saw my primary and all was good. He projected what would happen past chemo.[7]

On August 20 I was scheduled for a PET scan and CT scan of the eyes and neck to the thighs. These tests were done with contrast and required the twenty-four-hour prep because of that iodine-dye reaction. Veins on the top of the hand were assaulted. The first tech got in with the first prick, but it hurt for quite a while. I thought I was set for the CAT scan, but alas, when they tried to inject the dye, it felt like shredded glass and needles. The needle had to be pulled. A nurse was on each hand, trying to find a vein. Three collapsed, one blew (that really hurt!), and the fifth attempt was successful. What an ordeal! This was a long day with lots of waiting for my husband.

Every six weeks I need an appointment to have the chest port flushed. My next meeting with the oncologist was in November. He said they would continue to monitor me and run tests for three years. If nothing showed up, after that period, I could be considered cured. So we take one day at a time, take time to smell the roses and praise God for every pain free breath we take. I am happy to report eyebrows are growing back, and I now have a covering of fuzz on my head. During the period of hair loss, would you believe the facial hair remained? Drat![8]

---

[7] "Come unto me, all ye that labor and are heavy laden, and I will give you rest" (Matthew 11:28).

[8] "And the peace of God which passeth all understanding, shall keep your hearts and minds through Jesus Christ" (Philippians 4:7).

Feelings

One day was filled with sadness. No happy thoughts came to mind. The following day was filled with gladness. Many hymns and choruses espousing praise and joy filled my heart—"Praise God from Whom All Blessings Flow," "Praise Him, Praise Him," "I've Got that Joy, Joy, Joy, Joy Down in My Heart," "How Great Thou Art," "Isn't He Wonderful?" "There Shall Be Showers of Blessing," to name a few. What a welcoming emotion following the doom and gloom of the day before.

At the height of my emotions, I penned the following letter:

My darling husband,

I awakened in the wee hours this morning my heart overflowing with my love for you. I was thinking how meaningless marriage vows are for so many. "For richer, for poorer, in sickness and in health."

We are now being tested, and you are proving yourself to be the ultimate soul mate. We haven't been able to share many private moments; besides, I could never say these things to your face without losing it. By now your eyes are probably filled with tears as are mine as I write. There are times we can best express our feelings through writing. We have to *vent* so our heart doesn't break. It helps; it really does.

I shall try to be brief. Is that possible with your motormouth wife?

The challenge before us is great and a fierce battle looms before us, but I know we are up to the fight. You know I believe God is in our corner. I wish you could have faith as I do. What other source is omniscient, omnipotent, and omnipresent? A bulwark in the time of storm that never gives way? I hadn't intended to include the former thoughts, but the words just flowed out of my pen.

I can't begin to tell you how much you mean to me. You have seen me through trials and tribulations with my parents, my work, our disagreements, etc. We were never promised a *rose garden*, but we have spent many times where we gained rich rewards of strength from supporting each other.

Your visits and your phone calls uplift my spirit. I know I don't begin to understand how hard this whole situation is on you, my doctor husband, with so much knowledge, my controller and helpmate who cannot direct this scenario. How I wish you could be spared this ordeal. Were our positions reversed, I don't know if I could be as strong as you.

We are blessed with many loving, caring friends. Although we feel we can deal with all this alone, do not be ashamed, too proud, or whatever to take advantage of their support. Do not hesitate to unburden your worries and concerns with those you trust—it is a mental catharsis and will free you from this onerous load you are carrying.

I could ramble on and on, but I think you get the gist of what I am trying to say. [9]

Forever and beyond my love,
Your wife,
Elaine xxxooo

---

[9] "Weeping may endure for a night, but joy cometh in the morning" (Psalm 30:5b)

Encounters

Included here are highlights of some of the people I met along the way.

I discovered that no two stories are alike, even if they may share some features.

Megan was my first charge nurse; she made me comfortable and tended to my needs—a great gal.

Ron, age fifty-seven, was one of the housekeeping staff. The poor guy is allergic to disinfectant sprays and has to wear a mask. Married thirty-six years, he has eight children—the oldest is thirty-six, and the youngest, twenty-three, writes poetry.

Nurse Katrina received speech therapy for a lisp as a child. She remembers hating to be reminded by her mom when she had something to say. No trace of fronting is noted now.

Kehra majored in nursing as a grad student at Cedarville College. Cedarville is a church-related school, and I remember visiting with our church group eons ago. Had they offered speech and hearing therapy, I might have gone there.

Yvette's fifty-two-year-old husband is terminal. He was battling an unidentified cancer in his neck for over a year. His history sounded much like mine—scary. They went through all the tests and removed his tonsils in an effort to determine the etiology of the tumor. In the meantime, he had been complaining about his back. Apparently, the cancer wasn't isolated. Yvette believes God's will be done and said she would pray for me. How wonderful and caring people can be, even when tested to the utmost.

In speaking with a woman in the nourishment room, I learned about her sixty-one-year-old spouse who was diagnosed in 2004. She named the type of cancer, but I never heard of it. Her husband had surgeries and chemo and was in remission, but the cancer has returned and he hasn't been responding to the chemo. How many manifestations of this horrible disease are there anyway?

One of the nurses' aides noted my bandaged neck and compared symptoms and tests run. She had discovered a small lump a few months ago. They are looking at parotid involvement because she has difficulty swallowing. She recovered from a TIA a short while back—a slight mouth shift to the left is the only residual indication of neurological involvement I could see.

As I was waiting for the PET scan, I met a fifty-two-year old woman on a cart; her English was very limited, and a friend was with her to act as interpreter. They were from Burma. The conversation was interrupted by a technician. He said I was not supposed to use my throat muscles in talking for it interfered with the infusion I just had. I must now be resigned to silence—the death knell for one who loves to talk! They brought me some magazines to help pass the time.

Speaking with a couple, I learned the husband has multiple myeloma that was diagnosed two years ago. He went through a series of tests followed by different treatments including chemo. He had just had a stem cell transplant from his own harvested cells.

As I was making my turn around the quadrangle, I met Diana and her spouse. She had been diagnosed a couple of years ago. Her progress has been up and down. Chemo depleted her strength and energy, and she had gone home to recover. She was beginning to feel better and returned for more chemo. They just had a stem cell transplant. One of my team doctors came up to us and remarked on the song she heard about from other team members—"National Embalming School." I wasn't sure how the lyrics would go over with Diana, but she got a hoot out of it and wanted a copy. It is indeed a small world. Diana had been a nurse in the Mayfield school system, where I taught my first six years. She was acquainted with

Judy, my coworker. We had a nice chat. So many people, so many stories.

Elsa, fifty-three-year-old from Niles, spent five months on a cot in her husband's room while he was being treated in the hospital. He was diagnosed with blood cancer. After the placement of three different ports, the final one has worked for two months—light at the end of the tunnel, hopefully. I shared "Fragments" and cancer writings. We hugged and wished each other health. Later Elsa came to my room and asked me to sign my book, *Innocence Lost*.[10]

Gladys, a caregiver from Alabama, has stage one myeloma. She never told anyone about her symptoms and fears it is in advanced stages. She walks very slowly and uses a cane. She said it hurt to walk. She thanked me when I gave her copies of "Fragments" and "Invasion."

On one of my walks, I met Rabbi Saul and his wife, Irina; she was diagnosed with breast cancer in January. They have a fourteen-year-old and a nine-year-old. She has been in and out of the hospital with chemo treatments and was going home that day. I promised to send them a card. Rabbi Saul gave me his business card if I needed anything. We wished each other well and a painless prompt healing.

A social worker is available to help a couple or significant other find convenient places to stay while undergoing treatment. One couple lives about an hour away from UH, and The Gathering Place found a nearby accommodation where they could stay and intermingle with others in similar circumstances.

What a story Linda shared about her niece and her experience at Petro. She's one of fifteen children. Linda decided to pursue a nursing career when she was frustrated by her inability to interrupt when her niece's doctor ineptly tried to explain the death of her full-term baby girl after she fell during a big snowstorm. From the emergency room, Mary was sent to one hospital and then transferred to Petro. She waited twenty-four hours before they did anything—something

---

[10] "But thanks be to God, which giveth us the victory through our Lord Jesus Christ" (1 Corinthians 15:57).

about the baby being separated from the mother in the placenta, no full explanation. The doctor referred to the infant girl as *it*; she had been given a name. The young mother was told, "You're young, you already have two children, and you can have more." One can't help but wonder what he would have told his wife given the same set of circumstances. We realize doctors cannot become emotionally involved, or they would crack up. Nonetheless, some form of humanity should be displayed. A travesty—how many sad tales are out there?

Is it a *he* or a *she*? You have a fifty-fifty chance of getting it right, and within a span of five days, I missed two out of two. How's that for a record?

I was waiting for an X-ray at university, and transport left the cart sideways to the TV. I could not look at the screen without getting a crick in my neck. Also waiting for an X-ray was a teenager (outpatient). When I commented about the positioning of the cart, the mother directed her youngster to relocate it. We started talking, and the child said he was in for an X-ray of the head. He had been attacked by a gang. "You have to stay away from people like that" was my sage advice.

"What are *you* in here for?" asked the teen. I told him about the lymphoma, and he asked if he could feel it. I had no objection, so he gently touched the mass. I attempted to explain the disease and mentioned the lymph system. This child had no clue about the different body systems. Wouldn't you think becoming familiar with your body would be a required subject available to all in the schools? By my use of pronouns, you know I thought I was speaking to a boy. My only excuse is I was not wearing my glasses and everything was blurry. When the nurse came for me, she said, "You know, that was a girl you were talking to."

Oops. "Was I gender specific as I was talking?"

"You were, but I don't think she minded."

On one home hiatus, we were at Waffle House, and my husband and I noted an adult with his back to us. He was wearing one of those bandana hankies over his head. Anthony said in jest, "Could we have your head covering?" He proceeded to remove the scarf covering my baldness and surgery stitches. I said, "I always wondered how you gals tie up those scarves." When we walked around to the front of the booth, I discovered I had been talking to a guy—missed again. He didn't act offended, thankfully. He was there with his girlfriend—she had graduated from college, and he was enrolled. He showed me how he did the head cover—I've been practicing, and I think I've got the hang of it.

Back in the hospital, Nurse Kerry caught me writing in the semi dark during the night shift and asked what I was writing. I shared my encounter with Margaret and told her my intentions for sharing my story. We had an extensive exchange of information that was very rewarding.

Joanne turned out to be a precious sister of the heart—what tenuous thread reached out and bound us together? As strangers, we met on our walks—Joanne wore a mask because she was neutropenic at the time of our first encounter. She was a seasoned veteran concerning matters relating to cancer and its treatment; I was the new kid on the block. Our eyes met, and God's magic touch somehow drew us together. Our song is "Only Believe." Where did you come from? What is your background? Who cares when all is said and done? The importance of life is what we make of it—enduring encounters and lasting friends. Friendships may arise for a reason, for a season or for a lifetime.

I had a surprise visit from Joanne in the morning. I discovered she too is a born-again Christian—what a bonding connection. I am ashamed I have monopolized our conversations thus far. I need to listen more and talk less.

Joanne and I have the same night duty nurse. When she came to deliver my meds, she found an empty bed. "She's escaped!" she thought. Then she remembered hearing me say I wanted a picture of Joanne and tracked me down.

On April 22 a young man from housekeeping came to pick up trash. I asked, "What's a nice boy like you doing in a place like this?"

He said, "I ask myself that every day." On further conversation he revealed he wants to be a mortician—naturally, I shared the "Embalming School" song. I asked if he would repeat that song to a cancer victim, and he said "No" emphatically. I guess it wouldn't be appropriate coming from a mortician, but it depends on the disposition or state of who you are talking to. Even though I've shared—not in a bad way, I think—I must curb my exuberance for that type of dark humor.

Marathon Man, a long-legged giant in neutropenic stage, nearly ran me down. I estimate he completes three to four rounds to my one—nonstop. When I commented on his speed, he said, "I'm younger than you are."

"You had to say that," I replied.

He rephrased his statement saying, "Well, I have longer legs." That explains it, more acceptable by far. He's evidently established a rigid routine. I caught him on the fly to hand him a "Fragments."

I called after him, "Look it over in your leisure. If you don't like it, please give it back rather than throwing it away." He noted my room number and said he'd do that.

Charlotte in housekeeping told me about her children. One daughter, a college graduate, writes poetry for the love of it. She has been told she could be published, but she hasn't gone that route. A thirty-three-year old daughter drives for RTA. She has taken a few classes and is single with no children. I suggested checking into the coast guard for a possible career. Note: my husband often advised young people to go into the service when they had no idea what they wanted to do in life.

Todd walked with his wife, Marie. She was seventy-two years old, a smoker, and was recently diagnosed with lung cancer. It had metastasized, which is not a good sign.

Rowena asked, "Have you named your pole? I call mine Brother Man." She recently had a kidney biopsy. As she seemed to be a kindred spirit and exhibited right-brain learning tendencies like me, I gave her a copy of "Fragments."

I had not thought about naming my pole and considered Albatross as appropriate, for it was a pain to be tethered to it. But no, it is really my friend and is here to help me. Other possibilities flooded my mind, and I settled on Sunshine. So many happy songs are associated with sunshine—"Heavenly Sunshine," "Sunshine on My Shoulder," "Sunshine on a Cloudy Day," "There Is Sunshine in My Soul Today."

Ron and Nancy identified the quadrangle walk as a race track—thirty-three cards to a lap. They named each section; he had a red car on his IV pole. Nancy likes cats and cat stories. The more we talk, the more we find we have in common.

Steve walked with Susan. About six years ago, she was diagnosed with breast cancer. It has metastasized into the brain, and she suffers short-term memory lapse. I learned Susan has two daughters and is fighting to survive. She is also a born-again Christian.

Quentin, a junior in high school, wants to be a muscleman.

One of the attendants suggested taking a few masks home with me when walking around outside—excellent idea. Isn't communication great?

We met Katrina a number of times, either checking in or checking out of UH—she has brain cancer. Returning my food tray, I saw her on a transport cart. "How are your headaches?" I inquired.

"After my lumbar puncture, they have been getting worse—that's why I'm back in. I was readmitted at 5:00 a.m. They think there may be leaking of spinal fluid. Maybe they can seal it off with my blood." Such suffering, poor child. She is only seventeen.

Linda is a true prayer warrior. She shared the following: To have healthy happy plants, they require rain or water and sunshine, but they also need to be talked to, sung to, played music to, and be introduced to other plants in order to thrive. Don't people fit into a similar pattern?

I was looking for Christina and accidently walked into Jeff's room. He was diagnosed with non-Hodgkin's lymphoma, and an infection from his IV had swelled his arm. He anticipated going home, and now he was stuck here until the infection cleared. I tried to cheer him as he was very depressed.

Kevin listens to heavy metal as he does his walk-around.

A Harley man was at UH to visit his wife. When I noticed the logo on the back of his shirt, I mentioned my Harley poem. I gave him "Fragments," and he stopped by later and said he appreciated the tribute to veterans as he's a Vietnam War vet.

I met a young man transported here. He has been going through kidney dialysis for eight years and was waiting to be called for his treatment. He looked so sad, I gave him "Fragments" to help pass the time. He was shy and reluctant to talk. I forgot I had my mask on and he probably thought, "Who's this weirdo?"[11]

Moe stopped to say they were going home to W VA; she'll be the caregiver. Jeff said they had been staying at Hope Lodge. Because of an infection, he previously spent many weeks at a Beachwood Motel.

A thirty-six-year-old clinical partner named Leaf visited me and shared quality time. I learned she had come up with an invention, but she found a patent would cost $600, out of reach for her pocketbook. She also has a book idea about relationships. When she mentioned her tendency to procrastinate, I told her it was one of my great flaws. I gave her a copy of "Fragments" and pointed out a poem titled "Procrastination." Leaf proved to be an avid listener as I told my story.

When Leaf's son was two and a half years old, he stuttered. As periods of dysfluency occurred, she fought to remain quiet and listen—she shed her tears in private. At the end of our visit, she said she was motivated to pursue her writing. Synchronicity strikes again!!

On one of my exercise jaunts, I met Steve. He wore a dinosaur-research shirt—interesting. When I was teaching, I acquainted

---

[11] "Verily, verily. I say unto thee, except a man be born again, he cannot see the kingdom of God" (John 3:3).

"That which is born of the flesh is flesh: and that which is born of the spirit is spirit" (John 3:6).

myself with dinosaur lore, for it was part of the second-grade curriculum. Steve said the pay is not great, but he enjoys his retirement job.

A young woman helped me remove a plate to reheat in the microwave. There are four girls in her family, and their forty-year-old mother was diagnosed with cancer. The family is rallying round, but the victim is having a difficult time dealing with her situation.

The night nurse came in and asked if I *wanted* my bed raised to the highest position. I hadn't noticed the change in bed height, but I knew I had a terrible time climbing in and out. Thank you, Nurse Linda.

Mara was wearing a mask and looked like an Arabian Princess. Eyeliner accented her lids, and mascara enhanced her eyelashes. She wore a coral dress with sparkly silver shoes and a scarf wound tastefully around her head—an angel and a circle pin were placed where the ends crossed. At the time of our encounter, her vivacious eyes revealed an indomitable spirit. She tries to look nice for her young daughter. When she learned of her cancer diagnosis, she had her head shaved and donated her hair to Wigs for Kids.

Her little daughter brought me a rainbow scarf to cover my baldness. Mara showed me some ways I could wrap the scarf around my head – the trick is to anchor the scarf behind the ears.

One patient strongly resembled Diane Keaton, the movie star. She was dispirited and angry—she feels she wasn't given a definitive diagnosis or an understandable plan of treatment. She has been trying to talk with her doctor, without success. She reads the Bible daily and prays, but she does not feel comforted—she is tired and weak. Is this her testing time?

The music therapist stopped by, and I showed her the CD Guy made that included "Victory"—adapted from my original "On Top of Old Baldy." I gave her copies of "Fragments," "Invasion," and "On Top of Old Baldy." Caitlyn said she could put my poems to music but later decided it would work better if I read the words aloud, and the music-therapy group would add a musical background. She asked if I'd be willing to participate in an NBC telecast about music therapy on Thursday. I said I would if I'm still here. Wow! Will wonders ever cease?

After I wrote about reactions of strangers, a dear nurse friend posed a question. Had I noticed how people responded when they learned I had cancer? I shared my perceptions, which were positive. She said, "Oh, I thought they might pull back to avoid any contact."

Perhaps some folks reacted in this way, but I was unaware of it. I can't help but wonder if my perception stemmed from my focus. What we look for, we will find. Stress the positive, and it will be foremost. Stress the negative, and it will be prominent. I believe many conclusions emanate from our state of mind.

I now observe actions of people I meet. Noting a covered, obviously bald head, one assumes some kind of cancer or treatment is in progress. I tend to adopt this attitude myself, failing to recognize there are many other reasons people are bald. It seems facial expressions tend to be more kindly; occasionally, encouraging words are offered—often repeated are "I'll be thinking of you" and "You are in our prayers." How can strangers who don't even know my name offer prayers on my behalf? Nonetheless, God knows who I am, doesn't he?

A Special time with Susan, My Violin Teacher

Susan shared a visit to the Friends Church. She anticipated a quiet, controlled service. At first she was amazed by how huge the assembly was. There was a band, loud responses from the congregation, and hand waving—not at all what she expected.

She was thinking of instituting a music program to meet requirements of the homeschooled. A woman gave her a lead where about 130 children were involved. She received a call inquiring into instrument availability and price. In the course of the conversation, the woman asked if all her teachers were Christians. Susan said she really didn't know. After all, religion wasn't a focus in her music program. Then Susan said, "I've never been asked that question before." The woman replied, "That's what my gynecologist said when I asked him." Susan was in a quandary, trying to make a connection, when the lady continued, "I wouldn't go to a gynecologist who wasn't a Christian and pro-life." Isn't that something?

Anne, a Sister of the Heart

Anne's visit overlapped with Susan's. She had gone to lunch with her sister, who accompanied her. We had a beautiful visit. The best gift one can give another is their time.

Another sister of the heart sent me a bookmark with a "Victory Torch" raised on the front. How uncanny is that? I make my fingers form a V sign to fellow cancer sufferers I pass. V is our victory symbol against all odds. Coincidence, you might say. "Nay," I reply, "'tis God inspired."

The accompanying verse I must share is Romans 8:37–39: "In everything we have won more than a victory because of Christ who loves us. I am sure that nothing can separate us from God's love—not life or death, not angels or spirits, not the present or the future, and not powers above or powers below."

Spiritual Side

When I was eight years old, I asked Jesus to come into my heart. From that time a new nature filled my soul with guidance from the Holy Spirit. My desire was to follow Jesus, and when confronted with controversial situations, I asked, "What would Jesus do?" Being human, I still made many wrong choices, and when I confessed my sins, God forgave me. Up until the time I married, I was active in my church. After that time, I did not change my beliefs, but I no longer went to church. My life changed greatly with the cancer diagnosis, and God revealed himself from the onset. Even though I neglected him for forty-two years, he remained faithful to me. How blessed I am.

In "The Mass," I had a mysterious visit from a stranger.

Before treatment started I met Margaret.

The week following tests and surgeries, I presented a bald head, dark bruising under my eyes, and a large bandage on my neck. My husband was visiting with a woman in the whirlpool of a local resort. I wanted to get a copy of my poems from the car to share with her and took a shortcut around the hot tub to access the door to the outside. Margaret, sitting on a pool lounger, was working on a paper—cut off at the pass! I saw the word *accommodation* on the top of one of the sheets and deduced she was connected to special education in some way and mentioned I was a retired speech-language pathologist. A conversation ensued, and the breadth and depth of the subject was above my head. We visited for a time, and then she pointed to my head and bruising with a questioning look. I explained what I was going through and mentioned I was fortunate for many people were praying for me. "Praying to who?" she asked.

"To God," I responded.

"What God?" She continued, "Allah, Mohammad, who?" At this point I was at a loss, for I did not want to offend her. I attempted to explain that I respected the beliefs of others and my own position. "What did God put into every human being that is unique to each individual, and even he cannot surmount it?" Is that a loaded question or what? I was put on the spot and threw out typical responses, but I was floundering.

I presented my ideas, and she gave periodic encouragement by saying, "You're getting close."

I said, "I just cannot come up with the answer."

"Yes, you can," she responded with confidence. I was not so sure. "Anyone can share the answer, but the full impact of the word only comes across when you arrive at the answer yourself. I leave you with that question. Once the answer is revealed to you, you will wonder why it didn't enter your head before." As this astounding woman spoke to me, she discouraged interruptions. "I only have a short time with you and must finish without interruptions." As she talked I kept trying to insert my own insights, and she frustrated me by continuing to put her fingers to her lips—shushing me. I felt handcuffed and a bit resentful, not being allowed to speak my piece. She said, "Our time together is short, and I must tell you all I have to say." I understand now we need to learn to listen without interrupting—a hard thing for me. When she finished, she asked if she could pray with me—I was blessed indeed.

I've decided I have been hiding too long. From ages eight to twenty-five, I was open about where I stood concerning my commitment to God. After I married I experienced a different lifestyle, and my spiritual side retreated—shame on me!

Am I on a *high* here? I don't recognize myself at this point, nor do I understand my openness to declare my relationship with my heavenly Father.

How strange that little in my former writings had anything to do with God—and yet some bits and pieces emerged in the writing of "Innocence Lost" and "Fragments." It's so mind-boggling, I cannot comprehend it. Whether or not I survive this ordeal is immaterial. I pray my story will ease the way for another—that is my greatest wish.

We can never undo what has been done—we can only move on, live, profit from lessons learned, avoid making the same mistakes over and over. Without God's help, it is impossible. "Who is this God?" you might question. I only have my own answer—you must find yours; it is an entity outside yourself.

I never thought I'd have a spiritual reawakening after forty-one years. Will God's great wonders never cease? I never forgot my religious convictions and beliefs, but I had ceased to practice them. All spiritual commentary is a result of my renewed commitment to God.

I disrespect Satan worship; it's pure evil. I do not know where that thought came from.

I naively posed the following question to my team, "Are you a creationist or an evolutionist?" Fools rush in—you know the rest. As an afterthought, I wish I had not put them on the spot.

Note to self: I tend to jump in like a bull in a china shop, heedlessly throwing out words of advice—learn to be more circumspect.

There is no life without death—for everything there is a season. I believe God inspired the men who wrote his Word. We read the original sin of our disobedience was passed down from our first generation—Adam and Eve. When God breathed life into Adam and Eve, he gave them something unique—freedom of choice that even he in all his power could not overcome. God did not create robots; he created living, breathing souls. When you recognize that extra ingredient instilled in you, all will become clear. The blinders will fall away, so simple yet so elusive—a wisp of smoke. Seek and ye shall find. Ask and it shall be opened unto you.

PHOTOS

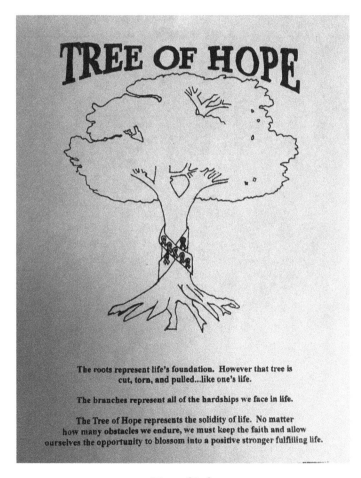

Tree of Life

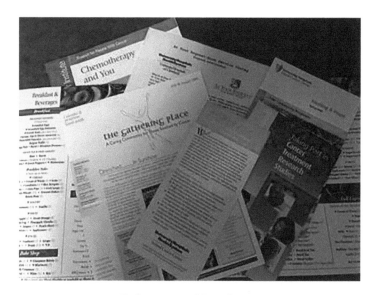

Informational Brochures

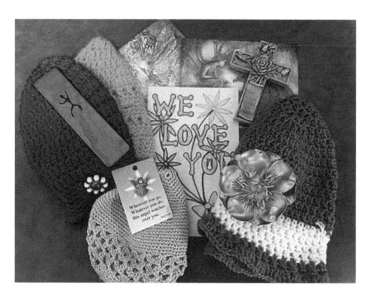

Chemo Caps, Cards, Survivor Bookmark,
Angel Pin and Mark 10:27 Cross

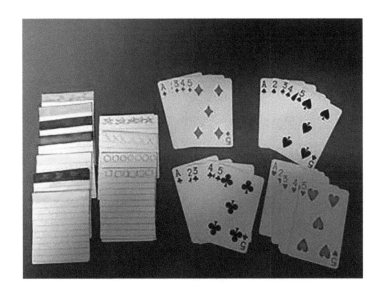

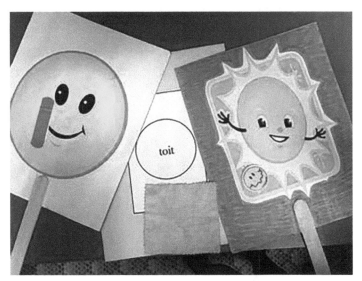

Quadrangle Counters, Mood, Aroundtoit
Symbol, Pole Banner, Prayer Cloth

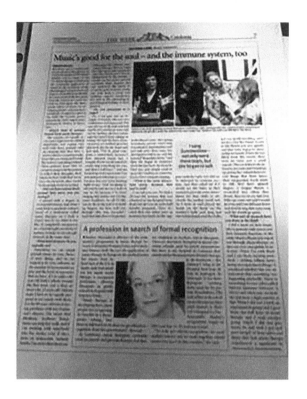

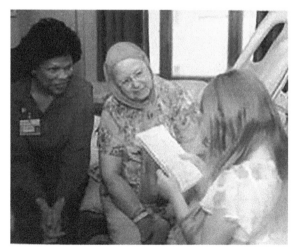

Music Therapy article – Music as Medicine

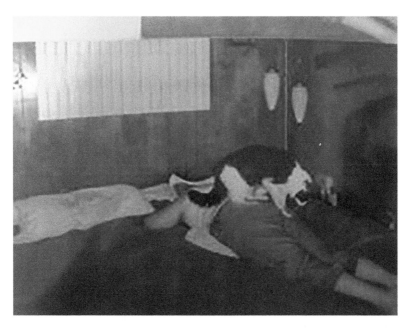

Domino my masseuse cat

My hospital life for 5 months

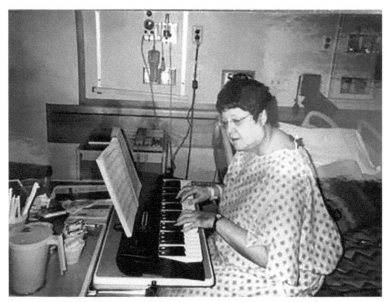

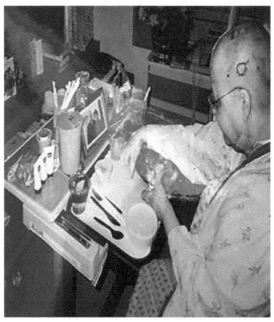

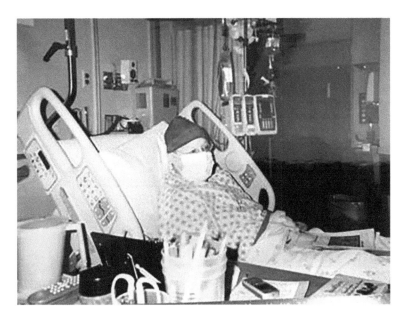

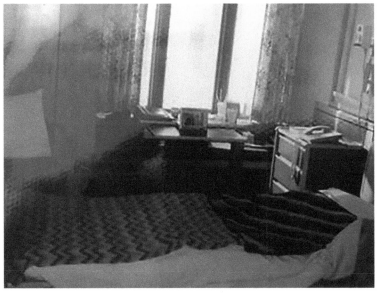

Random Thoughts

W hence come forth these random thoughts that make me restless until I write them down? Dustin, a respiratory therapist, came into my room at 4:15 a.m. looking for a piece of equipment. He asked if I were all right or needed help. I assured him all was well, but I needed to write down these random thoughts lest they escape me. "Weird, I know," was my explanation.

"Nothing weird," his reply.

I try to be objective in my outlook; however, I tend to believe my way of thinking is not that different from other human beings'. I failed to factor in that a solution for me might not be feasible for another.

In this place we are racing against death—dragging our heels, arming our defenses, bringing in the big guns, knowing full well many good guys will fall. Our goal is surviving—defeat this rebel sprung from our bodies and run amok encroaching on the terrain of body systems and turning them into barren wasteland.

Fortifying defenses are up, my army is prepared to fight the rebel cancer cells; we shall overcome.

A bald head is something else. I wasn't prepared for the sensation of hair loss. It feels moist. Covering my naked head made me more comfortable, yet I still have sensations from the recent port implant. I'm opting for mom's knit square and a head scarf to offset the unfamiliar *coldness*. Wigs do not appeal to me at this point. We shall see down the line. Cap and scarf coverings work well.

Coping—how to hygienically deal with a head losing hair. A male aide introduced me to the shampoo cap. What a great invention!

In a thank-you note to Gretchen, I wrote, "Who would have thought your Christmas hat would become a treasure covering my bald head at night? The pleasant-scented soothing creams are most welcome."

I see a caregiver, spouse, or friend—lines of worry crease their foreheads as they try to act normal, dying inside for their loved one, inconsolable, unable to share their pain or take it upon themselves if they could.

Where does our natural, untrained talent spring from in the areas of art, music, writing, mathematics, and inventions? I believe it is God-given. Look at the savants—what scientific logic can explain their uncanny ability when they appear to have little cognitive association?

It has to be a nightmare! I am in a terrible dream where people are walking round and round a quadrangle—some have IV poles, some bald-headed, some are in need of assistance. Zombies—they seem like the living dead, some stepping along, others hesitant, yet others dragging with frequent stops at rest benches placed along the way. Horror of horrors, *I am one of them! Masks cover some faces— some are jaunty, and others are weak and halting, pushing on.*

I choked when attempting to drink water in a reclining position. I am one who must be vertical to get pills down. Drinking from a water bottle helps some, but those horse-size tablets don't want to go down. More water and more water—swallow, swallow, please go down. Pills must be forced down so they can do their thing. Each medication is identified and I'm told its purpose, but my mind is too muddled to take it all in. I want to remember, but it escapes me—like chasing a rainbow, taunting but elusive.

As mass size decreases, so does pressure on the neck. Thank God the headaches diminished to an occasional dull thud. I don't need to cry uncle yet.

Topic—Cancer

The outside world might talk about it, write about it, paint about it, sing about it, do research on it, dream about it, imagine it, campaign about it, raise money for it, donate money to it, join support groups, volunteer for it, teach about it, preach about it. Go through it? No way, not voluntarily!

I can smell sweat from damp armpits—didn't get to deodorant today.

Daily mouth care is vital to discourage formation of ulcers and sores. Who needs those?

My 2007 Christmas update told of our rutted existence of primarily eating and sleeping, but recognizing how fortunate we were to have a place to eat nourishing food, teeth to chew, digestive system intact, sleeping in a clean bed, and having shelter. How much we take for granted. Be forewarned against complacency.

Thoughts keep spinning out—radiating in different directions, unrelated, where do I take them? Into yet another book, too much to take it all in, yet I feel all is not relative to this title. Sort and sift—my job or another's? It's too strange.

We view a victim in the mirror trapped in another dimension—behold the participant. A loved one outside is beating at the bars, unable to reach the victim—behold the spectator.

Life can be likened to a bowling game—let the pins fall as they may.

An outside view—life seems to be going on around you. We're in a time warp, going nowhere on treadmills, isolated except when visited from the outside and tuned in to the media.

Do we desire to keep connected, or do we withdraw to our individual struggles?

Nobody wants to be told what to do. Even though we know this, why do we continue in our attempts to influence others to our way of thinking? Hmmmm.

Having typical characteristics of the right-brained learner, I relate whole to part. Give me a whole anything, and I'll readily take it apart. God is challenging me to use the left side of my brain—given parts, assimilate into the *big picture*. Each isolated encounter or revelation eventually interacts—*astounding*.

Healing old wounds, must reconnect, don't revisit past hurt. The time is now, the future is before us, dwelling in the past is nonproductive.

Give me the words. In our hearts we feel so many things; putting those emotions into words is difficult.

Ever see one of these? Note illustration. What we see is a round to it. Being of a literal mindset, I didn't get it without an explanation. How many times do we put things off, saying "I'll get around to it"? Guilty as charged. The time is now, such a precious commodity and how we waste it—guilty again. I am one of the biggest procrastinators ever.

When engaging in conversation, remember there is a natural resistance to any fabric that contains even a hint of judging or negativity. Don't be judgmental. Do be open-minded and accepting. Ask permission—"Do you mind if I share something with you?" Present facts, not opinions. How to convey useful thought-provoking info so it's palatable—a spoonful of sugar helps the medicine go down.

If a title isn't appealing, you're not interested.

Thomas Edison: I have not failed 999 times. I have found 999 ways that won't work.

Murphy's Law: If things can go wrong, they will.

Brannigan's law: Murphy was an optimist.

It Could Happen to You

Ellen Blackhart

There are things we encounter in our lives that we do not choose, but we have to just pick up our cross and go on—*one day at a time*. Most likely we will need a lot of help—we cannot go it alone.

On October 3, 2005, the day after my eighty-second birthday, I was in the doctor's office to hear the result of my biopsy. It was lymphoma (non-Hodgkin's). I remember thinking—I had no pain whatsoever in my groin area, so how could this be? I had cancer?

After the surgery comes the fun part—so many treatments. I had eight CAT scans, three PET scans, four chemos, followed by a Neulasta shot the following morning. There was Prednisone and four series of Rituxan treatments, which consisted of a treatment each Tuesday for one month and repeated in six months, making it sixteen in all. My next CAT Scan will be on October 6, 2008.

When going through the treatments and procedures, one cannot help thinking about the gifted doctors, nurses, technicians—all the help involved. They all have to be commended. God bless them all!

And there are the many prayers said and done by your precious and loving family and friends. That also plays a tremendous part in your ongoing recover.

Hail cancer survivors!

Definitions

Antigen:

Any part of a molecule capable of being recognized by the immune system. The immune system responds by producing antibodies that bind to the antigen.

Atypical Lymphocytes:

Lymphocytes that become large as a result of antigen stimulation. Typically, they can be more than thirty millimeters in diameter, with varying size and shape.

Biopsy:

A medical test commonly performed by a surgeon, interventional radiologist, or an interventional cardiologist involving sampling of cells or tissues for examination. It is the medical removal of tissue from a living subject to determine the presence or extent of a disease. The tissue is generally examined under a microscope by a pathologist and can also be analyzed chemically.

Burkitt's lymphoma:

A rapidly growing type of non-Hodgkin's lymphoma, first described in Africa where it may present as a cancer of the facial bones; in other countries, it usually affects the abdomen. It requires immediate treatment and is uncommon in western countries.

Central venous access port:

A small device placed under the skin in order to provide easy and ready availability to a vein.

Chemo:

Treatment of a disease by chemicals that kill cells, specifically those of microorganisms of cancer. In popular usage, it will usually refer to drugs used to treat cancer or the combination of these drugs into a standardized treatment regimen.

CHOP chemotherapy:

A lymphoma treatment that includes three medicines delivered through an IV and Prednisone in a pill form. One cycle takes five consecutive days.

CT or CAT scan (computed tomography):

A technique for imaging body tissues and organs resulting in a cross-section of the body at any level from the head to the feet.

Cytology:

A department that deals with the study of cells, their structures and functions, examination of cells obtained from body tissue, or fluid to establish if they are cancerous cells.

Differentiation:

Cells that change into specialized cells in aiding the development of tissues and the organs.

Digestion:

A process of breaking down ingested foods that can be absorbed into the blood and utilized by the body.

ENT specialist:
One who focuses on medical and surgical care for problems associated with ear, nose, and throat. ENT specialists also provide surgical care for head and neck disease.

Growth:
An increase in the size of a number of cells or an increase in the size of each individual cell.

Mass:
A growth usually assessed by measuring mass or volume and size.

Medical Personnel:
Attending physician
- Has ultimate responsibility for care during hospital stay
- Identified by the green stripe on ID badge

Licensed physician
- Training to become specialized in a specific area of medicine

Resident
- Responsible for day-to-day care
- Visits regularly to discuss condition

Intern
- Physician who has completed medical school in training

Physician assistant (PA)
- Has a bachelor or master's degree with advanced training in obtaining histories and performing physicals
- Supervised by an attending physician

Medical students
- Closely supervised by licensed physicians

Registered nurse (RN)
- Assess, monitor, plan, implement, evaluate nursing care for each patient

Primary nurse or relationship-base nurse
- Meets once a day to coordinate care and information needs

Clinical nurse specialists (CNS)
- Advanced practice nurses
- Consults on wound care, emotional support, pain control, trouble shoots problems, anticipates complications and helps to prevent them

Continuing care coordinators and case managers (an RN)
- Work with you, your family, your primary nurse, and the health care team to develop a plan for care after hospital discharge

Nursing care assistants (NCA)
Clinical partners (CP)
Clinical technical assistants (CTA)
Nursing assistant I
- In training and supervised by an RN
- Routine clinical tasks and daily activities

Secretary
- First responder to call light

Transfers request to responsible party

Methotrexate:

This is used to treat diseases associated with abnormalities and rapid cell growth such as tumors. Methotrexate in higher doses can cause adverse reactions. The most frequent are mouth sores, stomach upset, and low white blood counts. It can be toxic to the liver and bone marrow.

MRI (magnetic resonance imaging):

A test that clearly shows soft tissue or organs without the use of X-ray.

MUGA scan (multigated acquisition scan):

A test that uses a series of X-ray pictures to look at the chambers and blood vessels of the heart.

Neutropenia:

A lower than normal number of blood neutrophils, a type of white cell. A patient is susceptible to infection during this period.

Ommaya:

A device implanted under the scalp that is used to deliver anti-cancer drugs to the cerebral spinal, the fluid surrounding the brain and spinal cord.

Oncology:

A branch of medicine that studies benign and cancerous tumors, determining and understanding their development, diagnosis and treatment, and prevention.

PET scan (positron emission tomography):

A test that shows the difference between normal and abnormal tissues in the body.

PH levels:

PH levels of the blood or other key bodily fluids fall out of optimal PH range due to adverse metabolic or respiratory conditions. The human body goes through a variety of adjustments to try to correct the acid or alkaline imbalance.

If the body is too alkaline, a condition called alkalosis results. Conversely, an overly acid condition results in acidosis. Checking urine pH is one way doctors look for imbalances in the pH levels of the body. Testing blood pH levels is another option.

Responsiveness:

Reacting to chemo and drugs put into the body, detecting changes internal and external, and a reaction to that change.

Rituxan infusion:

Healthy B cells help your body fight infection. But in NHL, B cells become cancerous and form tumors. Rituxan targets B cell tumors. It also targets healthy B cells and leaves most other types alone. Used on its own or in combination with chemo, there are side effects. Fever, nausea, chills, itching, hives, cough, headache, sneezing, tightness, throat irritations, and shaking may occur with immunotherapy.

Twelve body systems:

Skeletal
Muscular
Integumentary/skin
Respiratory
Circulatory
Nervous
Urinary
Lymphatic
Digestive
Endocrine
Reproductive
Immune

Warthin's tumor:

A benign growth that forms in the salivary glands.

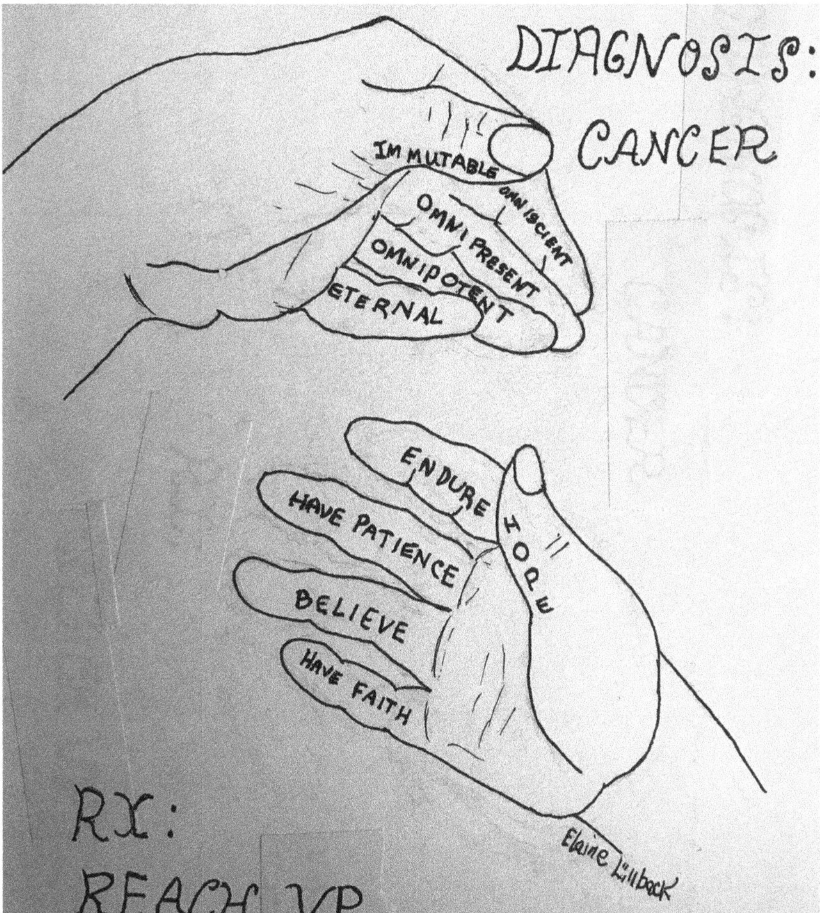
DIAGNOSIS:
CANCER
IMMUTABLE
OMNISCIENT
OMNI PRESENT
OMNIPOTENT
ETERNAL
ENDURE
HOPE
HAVE PATIENCE
BELIEVE
HAVE FAITH
RX:
REACH UP
Elaine Lillback

Author's Note

D iagnosis Cancer has been sitting on the shelf since 2008. I had discombobulated stacks of scribbled notes I wrote while hospital bound. Sorting through the piles of material was overwhelming. I presented the project to my dear friend Cathy, whom I consider my earth angel. Reluctant at first, she agreed to tackle the job, which involved umpteen title changes, numerous rewrites, and long hours of editing and sorting. With this huge undertaking, my everlasting gratitude goes to her—my collaborator, friend, and cowriter. Without her I could never have completed this book.

Closing thought:

We might lose the battle
but never the war;
United with Jesus,
to Heaven we soar.

The footnotes scattered throughout this book are taken from the King James Version [KJV] of the Bible. They appear sequentially and hold special meaning for me.

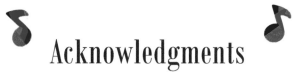 Acknowledgments

I would like to thank the following:

Primary doctor and ENT doctor
Team of doctors at University Hospital in Cleveland, Ohio
University nursing staff
Housekeeping staff
Robin
Family
Friends
All the above made a huge difference during my treatment and care.
Thank you from my heart and God bless.

Elaine M. Uonelli

About the Author

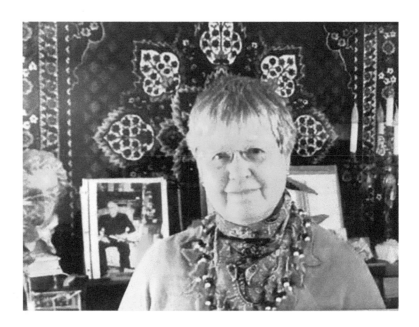

E laine currently resides in Perry, Ohio, with her three adopted cats. She is a self-published author of *Innocence Lost*, a novel, and *Fragments*, a collection of poems. Her hobbies include playing the piano and the organ, reading, writing, and adult coloring. A devout Christian, she wrote this book praying that the reader will find hope and comfort in the spiritual process one can go through when fighting this horrible disease.

To order a copy of

Diagnosis Cancer: I Can't Be Here,

go to Amazon.com or Barnes and Noble.com

CPSIA information can be obtained
at www.ICGtesting.com
Printed in the USA
LVHW070419170819
627914LV00005BA/61/P